DENNIS PANTUA

Writing Lives, Not Just Plans

The Compassionate Guide to Person-Centred Care Planning

First edition

This book was professionally typeset on Reedsy.
Find out more at reedsy.com

– A Letter to You

Dear Reader,

If you are opening this book, I already know something important about you: you care deeply about the quality of support people receive. You're not content with "good enough." You're curious, you want to learn, and you're willing to go further to make care more personal, more dignified, and more human. That makes you exactly the kind of person who can write a truly great, life-affirming care plan.

Contents

Introduction

Writing Lives, Not Just Plans

A care plan is never just paperwork. It is a person's story — written in a way that shapes how they are supported, respected, and valued every single day. Who writes the plan, and how they write it, matters deeply. And in this case, that person is you.

The fact that you are here, exploring how to write better plans, already shows your commitment to make care more compassionate and personal. Care plans are most powerful when they are co-produced — combining professional expertise with personal insight. Nurses, carers, managers, families, allied health professionals, and independent consultants all play a part. Yet it is your observations, your words, and your warmth that transform a plan from a checklist into a living story.

The Personality of the Writer Matters

You bring a plan to life when you:

- Write warmly, with compassion and curiosity.

- Use the person's own words wherever possible.
- Celebrate strengths, routines, belongings, and choices.

You flatten a plan when you:

- Use cold, copy-and-paste wording.
- Reduce a person to tasks, risks, and needs alone.

Traits of a Promising Care Plan Writer

- **Curious** – asks questions that uncover the "why."
- **Compassionate** – writes as if the person themselves will read it.
- **Observant** – notices the details that make someone unique.
- **Collaborative** – works alongside families, colleagues, and the person.
- **Reflective** – checks if wording promotes dignity and independence.
- **Empowering** – highlights abilities, not just difficulties.

Reflection for You

By reading this page, you have already begun the journey. Your intention, empathy, and professionalism are the strongest foundations for becoming the kind of care-plan writer who makes a genuine and lasting difference.

One

Why Care Planning Matters

Why Care Planning Matters

The Purpose of Care Planning

If you've worked in care for even a day, you've heard the words *care plan.*

For some, it brings a sigh — "more paperwork."

For others, a smile — "the backbone of good care."

The truth is that care plans are living, breathing stories, not forms.

They are essential tools for:

- **The person being supported:** to ensure they are truly seen, respected, and understood.
- **Carers:** to give confidence in delivering safe, consistent, and compassionate support.
- **Families:** to trust that their loved one is treated as an individual,

not a task.

A strong care plan makes the difference between:

- Being treated with dignity versus being seen as "just another resident."
- Having choice and control versus being told what to do.
- Feeling safe and supported versus being at risk of harm.

Think of the care plan as your roadmap:

- **Where we start:** strengths, life story, and needs.
- **Where we're going:** aims and outcomes.
- **How we get there:** plan of action.

Without this map, care becomes task-driven and inconsistent.
With it, care becomes personal, safe, and meaningful.

What a Care Plan Is

A care (or support) plan is a written document that:

- Describes the person's current strengths, abilities, and needs.
- Records life story, profession, personality, and character — not just medical facts.
- Captures what matters to them — their preferences, routines, and values.
- Provides clear, practical instructions for staff on how to support them.
- Identifies risks and explains how these will be managed safely.
- Includes personal belongings and equipment such as labelled

clothing, toiletries, hearing aids, or mobility aids.
- Is reviewed and updated as needs, wishes, or circumstances change.

In plain English: **a care plan is our written promise to provide care that is safe, personal, and full of dignity.**

The Legal and Regulatory Backbone

In the UK, care planning isn't just good practice — it's a legal requirement.

- **Care Quality Commission (CQC):** Inspects services against five key questions — Safe, Effective, Caring, Responsive, and Well-Led.
- **National Institute for Health and Care Excellence (NICE):** Provides evidence-based standards for best practice.
- **Mental Capacity Act (2005):** Protects people who lack capacity, ensuring decisions are made in their best interests using the least-restrictive option.
- **Deprivation of Liberty Safeguards (DoLS):** Ensure restrictions such as locked doors or supervision are lawful, proportionate, and regularly reviewed.
- These will be replaced by **Liberty Protection Safeguards (LPS)** to strengthen rights.
- **Confidentiality and Data Protection:** Care plans must be shared only with those who need the information for safe, compassionate care.

Bottom line: *if it isn't written in the care plan, it didn't happen.*

Supporting Independence and Positive Risk-Taking

One of the most powerful things a care plan can do is support independence — even when that means taking carefully managed risks.

Too often, risk is seen as something to avoid, but a life without risk can mean a life without freedom, joy, or growth.

A good care plan asks:

- *What matters most to this person?*
- *How can we support this safely?*

This is called **positive risk-taking.**

Example:

Instead of "John must not go out alone," write:

> *"John enjoys visiting the corner shop each afternoon. He values his independence but feels safer with company. One staff member will accompany him, walking at his pace. John will choose the items he wants and handle his own money, with support only if asked."*

This balances **safety with dignity.**

SMART Goals in Care Planning

Good outcomes are written using the **SMART** principle:

- **Specific** – clear and detailed.
- **Measurable** – progress can be tracked.
- **Achievable** – realistic for the person.
- **Relevant** – meaningful to their life.
- **Time-bound** – includes a timeframe.

Example:

"Mary will attend the weekly craft group (Specific) with staff support (Achievable) for the next 4 weeks (Time-bound), to build her confidence (Relevant), measured by attending at least 3 sessions (Measurable)."

Person-Centred vs Task-Centred Care

Task-Centred:

"Resident to be washed at 8 a.m."
"Resident to be hoisted into bed at night."

Person-Centred:

"Mary prefers a shower after breakfast using lavender body wash. She washes her face independently and asks for help only with her back."
"Amira usually goes to bed around 9 p.m. She uses a hoist for safe transfer and enjoys soft music while settling."

Task-centred care reduces people to routines.
Person-centred care celebrates individuality, dignity, and choice.

Reflection Corner

- Did your last care plan sound more task-centred or person-centred?
- Did it include details of the person's life story, character, and preferences?
- What small changes in language could make it more empowering?

Tips for Practice

- Write in the person's own voice.
- Write as if introducing the person to a new carer who truly wants to help.

Pitfalls to Avoid

- Generic, task-focused language.
- Omitting belongings, routines, or preferences.
- Failing to review or update the plan as things change.

Common Myths About Care Plans

- "They're just paperwork for CQC."
- → In truth, they *guide daily care* and *protect people.*
- "They're all the same."
- → Every plan should reflect a *unique individual.*
- "Once written, it's done."
- → Care plans are *living documents.*

Role-Specific Reflections

- **Carers:** daily guide for safe, confident care.
- **Family carers:** reassurance that individuality is respected.
- **Managers:** clear CQC evidence of person-centred practice; ensure staff are trained and competent.
- **Kitchen teams:** vital for allergies, culture, and food preferences.
- **Laundry / cleaning:** clothing and bedding routines uphold dignity.
- **Maintenance:** awareness of mobility and environmental needs supports independence.

- **Volunteers / visiting professionals:** insight into the person's story builds connection.

Quick Activity

Rewrite to person-centred language:

"Resident to be fed three times daily."

→ "I enjoy three meals a day. I like to take my time eating and prefer soup in the evening. Please sit with me and only assist if I ask."

"Resident to be hoisted into bed at night."

→ "I usually go to bed around 9 p.m. I need hoist support to transfer safely and enjoy soft music as I settle."

The One-Page Profile

A **One-Page Profile** captures the essence of a person on one page — quick to read, easy to use, deeply respectful.

It is not a legal requirement, but it demonstrates best practice and shows CQC inspectors that your service goes beyond minimum standards.

Example Format:

Important To Me:

"I like a cup of tea before I talk to anyone. Gospel music and my faith are important to me. I feel happiest with my grandchildren."

Important For Me:

"I need my inhaler twice a day. I feel safer with someone beside me on stairs. Please face me when speaking, as I wear hearing aids."

How Best to Support Me:

"Please knock before entering my room. Speak slowly and clearly. Encourage me to choose meals and don't rush me when I get dressed."

My Strengths and Abilities:

"I can wash my face and brush my teeth. I like folding laundry and reading the paper aloud."

My Aspirations and Goals:

"I'd like to visit the park weekly, try baking again, and join a local choir."

Quick Check:

- Does it sound like the person's own voice?
- Would they recognise themselves?
- Does it highlight strengths, not just needs?

Tip: Keep One-Page Profiles visible (with consent) — they should guide daily care, not sit forgotten in a folder.

Chapter Summary

Care planning is more than paperwork; it is the heartbeat of quality care.

It's about knowing the person, respecting individuality, and writing their story clearly so every team member can provide consistent, compassionate support.

A truly person-centred plan includes not only tasks and risks but also life story, profession, personality, belongings, and preferences.

It is a living agreement that protects rights, supports independence, and promotes dignity and joy.

Care planning is not paperwork — it is person-work.

Compliance Spine

- **CQC KLOE:** Safe (S2.1) | Effective (E1.4) | Caring (C1.1) | Responsive (R1.2) | Well-Led (W2.1)
- **NICE Quality Standard Check:** Does each care plan reflect the person's preferences, story, belongings, risks, and outcomes?

End of Chapter 1

Two

What "Person-Centred" Really Means

Seeing the Person Before the Task

When you're supporting someone at 7 a.m. on a busy shift, *person-centred care* means this:

- Seeing the person before the task.
- Fitting care around the individual — not forcing the individual to fit the care.
- Doing things *with* people, not just *for* them.
- Keeping people safe while enabling a life that feels like their own.

Ask yourself:

> *If you were receiving care, would your plan make you feel like a unique person — or like a checklist?*

The Four Pillars of Person-Centred Care

1. **Individuality** – No two people are the same, even with the same condition.
2. **Choice and Control** – Support people to make their own decisions wherever possible.
3. **Dignity and Respect** – Protect privacy, value beliefs, act with kindness.
4. **Independence and Safe Risk-Taking** – Encourage people to do as much as they can, safely.

Together, these pillars ensure care is both compassionate and empowering.

Seeing the Whole Person: Life Story, Personality, and Preferences

A truly person-centred plan brings together the person's:

- **Life story or profession:** Past roles help us connect — a retired nurse, a teacher, a builder.
- **Personality or character:** Match your approach — some prefer humour, others calm routine.
- **Values and beliefs:** Faith, culture, and personal principles shape care.
- **Preferences and routines:** From tea before talking to bedtime rituals — details create comfort.

Practice tip:

Ask, "What should we know about you so we can support you well?"

Routine-Led vs Person-Centred: Spot the Difference

Routine-Led:

> *"Breakfast is served at 7:30 a.m. for all residents."*
> *"Resident washed and dressed by staff."*

Person-Centred:

> *"James prefers tea and toast around 9 a.m. after reading the newspaper."*
> *"Maria chooses her outfit each morning; she needs help with buttons but prefers to brush her own hair."*

One approach makes people fit the system.
The other makes the system fit the person.

Why Person-Centred Care Is Non-Negotiable

- **CQC inspections:** Evidence of personalisation is required; copy-and-paste won't pass.
- **Quality of life:** People feel respected when preferences are honoured.
- **Staff confidence:** Clear, personalised guidance reduces guess-work.
- **Family trust:** Plans should reflect real lives, not generic wording.

Reflection Corner

- Was your last plan task-centred or person-centred?
- Did it include life story, character, and preferences?
- What language changes could make it more empowering?

The Power of Language

Cold, task-led:

> *"Resident requires assistance with feeding."*

Warm, person-centred:

> *"Mrs Patel enjoys meals with a small glass of wine. She eats independently but may appreciate staff checking whether she'd like support and time to finish at her own pace."*

Words can strip identity — or celebrate it.

Writing in the Person's Voice

First-person ("I"):

"I like a cup of tea before I talk to anyone in the morning."

"I prefer showers after breakfast and like lavender body wash."

"I need help with buttons when my arthritis is bad, but please let me choose my outfit first."

"I feel safer walking in the garden if someone is beside me. Please walk at my pace."

Professional third-person:

"Mrs Khan enjoys tea before starting her day and prefers quiet mornings."

"Mary prefers showers after breakfast, washes her face independently, and needs help with her back."

"John chooses his outfit each morning and usually needs support with buttons during arthritis flare-ups."

"Peter enjoys garden walks and feels safer with staff alongside him."

Best practice: Use both — the person's voice for identity, the professional's for clarity.

Balancing Safety and Independence

Risk-led:

> *"Do not allow Mary to walk without assistance."*

Person-centred:

> *"Mary enjoys short garden walks. She uses her frame and requires supervision for safety. Encourage this daily to support mobility and confidence."*

The second protects both *safety and dignity.*

Role-Specific Reflections

- **Carers and nurses:** Always ask before stepping in; offer choice even when help is needed.
- **Family carers:** Notice small routines — the favourite mug, the morning radio.
- **Kitchen teams:** Record how someone takes their tea, any allergies, cultural needs, and comfort foods.

- **Laundry and cleaning teams:** Clothing and linen preferences protect dignity.
- **Maintenance teams:** Environment matters — lighting, seating, rails, and signage affect wellbeing.
- **Managers:** Keep plans live; lead a culture of personalisation.
- **Volunteers and activities staff:** Reflect real interests — choir over bingo, if that's what matters.

Real-Life Practice Tip

Instead of saying, "Let me do that for you," try:

> *"Would you like me to help with your cardigan, or would you like to try first?"*

Small choices create big dignity.

Quick-Glance: Person-Centred in Practice

Ask – What are their preferences?
Listen – What truly matters?
Record – Capture details in the plan.
Respect – Honour identity, privacy, and choice.
Review – Update as lives change.

Activity – Rewrite in Person-Centred Language

"Resident to be given medication at 8 a.m."

→ "I usually take my tablets after breakfast with orange juice. Please check if I prefer water some mornings."

"Resident to attend activities twice weekly."

→ "I enjoy gardening club on Mondays and music afternoons on Fridays. Please encourage me, but respect if I prefer quiet time."

"Resident requires hoist transfer."

→ "I use a hoist for safe transfers. Explain each step and give me time to feel comfortable."

Person-Centred Planning Tools

Important To / Important For

Important To Me:

Having tea before speaking in the morning; spending time with grandchildren; going to church on Sundays.

Important For Me:

Taking medication at 9 a.m.; using hearing aids for communication; safe transport support.

Decision-Making Profile

How I decide: I need time to think; I prefer written options.

What others should know: I sometimes say "yes" to please — check with me twice.

How to support me: Offer choices in a quiet place; use simple language.

Doughnut Tool

Must do (non-negotiable): Give insulin at 8 a.m.; support hoist transfers safely.

Staff judgement/flexibility: Offer choice of clothing, activities, and meals.

Tip: Complete an "Important To / Important For" chart with someone this week — small details transform care.

Legal and Ethical Note – DoLS / LPS

Person-centred care includes lawful decision-making.

When a person's choices are restricted for their safety, this must be justified, proportionate, and regularly reviewed.

- **DoLS (Deprivation of Liberty Safeguards):** Protect people in care homes or hospitals who lack capacity to consent to certain care.
- **LPS (Liberty Protection Safeguards):** Will replace DoLS, expanding these protections across all care settings.

Plans should always show:

- That capacity was assessed.
- That the least-restrictive approach is in place.
- That any authorisation (DoLS/LPS) is clearly referenced and reviewed.

This demonstrates compliance with **CQC Safe (S2.1)** and **Caring (C1.1)** standards.

Key Takeaways

- Person-centred care sees the individual first, not the task.
- The four pillars: individuality, choice, dignity, and independence with safe risk-taking.
- Record life story, profession, personality, and preferences.
- Language matters — use the person's voice.
- Safe risk-taking is part of empowerment.
- Every role contributes to bringing the plan to life.

Chapter Summary

Person-centred care is the heartbeat of compassionate, high-quality care.

It shapes daily practice, language, and decisions — balancing safety with independence and dignity.

Plans must go beyond tasks to capture life story, personality, preferences, and aspirations.

Everyone — from carers to managers — plays a part in honouring the whole person.

Compliance Spine

- **CQC KLOE:** Safe (S2.1) | Caring (C1.1) | Responsive (R1.2) | Well-Led (W2.1).
- **NICE Quality Standard Check:** Does each plan show evidence of individuality, life story, choice, dignity, and independence?
- **Legal Note:** Restrictions on liberty are authorised under DoLS and, in future, LPS. Until LPS begins, services must fully comply with current DoLS requirements.

End of Chapter 2

Three

Why Start with Strengths

Starting with What's Strong, Not What's Wrong

Care planning can easily slip into describing what someone *cannot* do. Lists of risks and limitations can quietly take away a person's individuality.

The truth is, everyone has strengths. A strength may be a physical skill, emotional resilience, a treasured hobby, or even a warm sense of humour that lights up the room.

When we begin a care plan with C***urrent Strengths and Abilities,*** we change the story. Instead of defining someone by illness or dependency, we start with their humanity and potential.

Why Strengths Matter

Starting with strengths:

- **Boosts dignity and self-esteem:** people feel valued when abilities are recognised.
- **Encourages independence:** carers are reminded to step back and assist only where needed.
- **Shows the person, not the diagnosis:** focus moves from dementia or frailty to individuality.
- **Lifts staff morale:** writing about strengths feels hopeful and positive.
- **Promotes meaningful engagement:** activities grow naturally from hobbies and routines.
- **Supports safe risk-taking:** people continue doing what they can, safely.
- **Comforts families:** they see identity and ability continuing.
- **Demonstrates CQC compliance:** strengths-first planning is empowerment in action.

Every care plan should begin with:

> *"This is who I am, what I can do, and what makes me me."*

What Counts as a Strength

Strengths go far beyond physical ability. They include:

- **Physical:** walking with a frame, eating finger foods, washing upper body.
- **Cognitive:** recognising familiar faces, remembering favourite

songs, making simple choices.

- **Emotional:** calmness, humour, patience.
- **Social:** chatting with others, enjoying groups, greeting people warmly.
- **Life story and profession:** careers, family roles, achievements.
- **Personality and character:** optimism, independence, cheerfulness.
- **Preferences:** routines, hobbies, faith, clothing, and music.

Example

Deficit statement: "Resident unable to manage personal hygiene."

Strengths-based version:

> *"John washes his face and upper body independently and enjoys choosing his own toiletries. He requires support with harder-to-reach areas."*

Writing Strengths in Different Voices

Person's Voice ("I" statements):

"I enjoy folding small laundry items because it makes me feel useful."

"I can wash my face and upper body myself. Please help with my hair and back."

"I like to choose my outfit each morning, even if I need help with buttons."

Professional Voice:

"Mrs Khan enjoys folding small laundry items and takes pride in helping."

"John washes his face and upper body independently and needs support with hair washing."

"Mary selects her clothes daily and benefits from staff assistance with fastenings."

Best practice: Use both — person first, staff note second.

Recording Strengths in the Care Plan

Ask yourself:

- What does the person still do for themselves?
- What brings them joy or purpose?
- How can staff encourage or preserve these abilities?
- How can this be phrased positively and with dignity?

Putting Strengths into Practice

Recording strengths is only the beginning — *living them daily* is what matters.

Core principles:

- Encourage, don't take over.
- Notice and praise every effort.
- Build on familiar routines.
- Adapt rather than remove tasks.
- Balance safety with freedom and choice.

Role-Specific Examples

- **Carer:** Place the spoon in the person's hand before assisting.
- **Kitchen staff:** Provide finger foods to support independence.
- **Housekeeper:** Invite the resident to dust their bedside table with you.
- **Maintenance staff:** Allow a DIY-lover to hand you tools safely.

- **Family carer:** Encourage your loved one to stir the tea, even if you pour the water.

Top Tip:

> *Ask, "What's one step this person can still do themselves?" That's where independence lives.*

Language Matters

Deficit: "Resident is unable to mobilise safely without staff support." Strengths-based:

> *"Margaret mobilises safely with her walking frame and enjoys short garden walks, which help maintain her independence and wellbeing."*

Same fact — *different impact.*

Reflection Corner

Think of someone you support right now.

- What's one thing they can do independently?
- How could you phrase it positively in their plan?

Testimonies

Staff voice:

> *"I used to write that Mrs L 'can't dress herself.' Her daughter said,*

'Mum always picks her favourite scarf.'

I changed it to: 'Mrs L selects her scarf each morning and enjoys choosing colours. She needs staff help with buttons.'

That small change meant her daughter felt her mum's personality was seen."

Family voice:

"When I read Mum's plan and saw it start with her humour and hobbies, I felt relief. It showed me she was seen as a whole person."

Helen Sanderson Tool – Important To / Important For

Helen Sanderson's tools guide every plan with three questions:

1. Who is this person?
2. What's important *to* and *for* them?
3. How can we support them to live their chosen life?

This **Important To / Important For** chart balances joy and safety, helping us see both identity and wellbeing needs.

Important To Me:

- Having tea before speaking in the morning.
- Spending time with grandchildren.
- Going to church on Sundays.

Important For Me:

- Taking medication at 9 a.m.
- Using hearing aids for communication.

- Having safe transport support.

Person's Voice:

> *"It's important to me to have tea before talking in the morning. Please let me do that before giving my tablets."*

Professional Voice:

> *"Mary prefers tea and quiet time before conversation. Staff should respect this routine while ensuring medication is taken by 9 a.m. Offer tea first, then prompt medication kindly."*

Practice tip:

Keep both "to me" and "for me" statements visible to balance dignity and safety.

Mini-Audit Check

Does this section clearly show:

- What's important to *and* for the person?
- The person's own words alongside staff guidance?
- Strengths, routines, and abilities, not just needs?

This tool links directly with other person-centred resources such as the One-Page Profile, Decision-Making Profile, and Doughnut Tool.

Activity – Rewrite Deficits as Strengths

"Resident is incontinent."

→ "David uses the toilet independently during the day, needing only occasional reminders."

→ "Amira manages with pads and benefits from regular staff support."

→ "Peter uses continence products and tells staff when uncomfortable so his dignity is maintained."

"Resident cannot feed themselves."

→ "Linda eats finger foods independently and enjoys sandwiches at lunchtime."

→ "George uses an adapted spoon and, with guidance, manages most of his meal."

→ "Mary needs assistance with feeding but smiles and engages during mealtimes."

"Resident is confused."

→ "James forgets the day sometimes but follows his routine well with prompts."

→ "Margaret enjoys talking about childhood and recognises familiar staff; she benefits from reassurance when routines change."

→ "Frank is disoriented but responds positively to pictures, signs, and calm tones."

Key Takeaways

- Begin every care plan with strengths and abilities, never deficits.
- Include physical, cognitive, emotional, social, and life-story strengths.
- Use positive, empowering language.
- Encourage, adapt, and praise effort.
- Recognising strengths uplifts staff and reassures families.

- Safe risk-taking protects independence.
- Helen Sanderson's tools help balance identity and safety.

Compliance Spine

- **CQC KLOE:** Safe (S2.1) | Caring (C1.1) | Responsive (R1.2) | Well-Led (W2.1).
- **NICE Quality Standard Check:** Does each plan highlight abilities, life story, and personality using positive, empowering language?
- **Mini-Audit for Staff:** When reading this section, do you see a real person with individuality — or just a list of tasks?

End of Chapter 3

Four

Why Needs Must Be Clear

From Understanding to Action

If strengths show what someone *can* do, the **Identified Needs** section records where they *need support.*

This section isn't about highlighting weaknesses — it's about being *specific, clear, and compassionate.*

Think of it as a **bridge**:

It connects the person's current reality (what they find difficult) to the support actions that follow later.

A vague note like "needs help with meals" is not enough.

Staff need to know **what kind of help, when, why, and how.**

Clarity ensures dignity, safety, and consistency of care.

When Needs Are Vague, Care Becomes Inconsistent

Without clear direction:

- One staff member may sit patiently.
- Another may rush.
- Another may not help at all.

The result? Confusion — and sometimes risk.
A vague entry can lead to:

- A **missed medication**.
- A **fall** if equipment isn't used.
- A **meal skipped** or a moment of **embarrassment**.

Done well, identified needs build **safety, respect, and independence.**

The Three Dimensions of Need

Every care plan should recognise the full picture — not just medical needs, but emotional and social needs too.

1. **Health Needs:**

- Long-term conditions (e.g., diabetes, dementia, arthritis).
- Mobility, nutrition, continence, medication support.
- Pain management, skin care, pressure relief.

1. **Emotional Needs:**

- Support with anxiety, depression, or loneliness.

- Reassurance during personal care.
- Comfort after distressing events.

1. **Social Needs:**

- Family contact, friendships, community connections.
- Meaningful activities, hobbies, and routines.
- Faith, cultural, or spiritual practices.

Practice tip:
Ask yourself — *if this person had no family visiting, would their emotional, spiritual, and social needs still be recognised in their plan?*
(Aligns with **CQC E1.1** and **NICE QS13 – holistic assessment**.)

The Structure of a Good Need Statement

Every identified need should include:

1. **What** the need is.
2. **When** it arises.
3. **Why** support is required.
4. **How** staff should support.
5. **The person's preferences.**

Example
Vague:

> *"Resident needs help with medication."*

Clear:

> *"Sarah needs staff to remind her to take her tablets each morning with breakfast, as she forgets without prompting. She prefers water at room temperature and likes time to take tablets one by one."*

The Danger of Vague Entries

Vague:

> *"Resident needs support with meals."*

Person-centred:

> *"Anna requires prompting and gentle encouragement to eat. She needs staff to cut up her food and supervise due to a risk of choking. She prefers her main meal at lunchtime and enjoys a calm atmosphere."*

Person's voice:

> *"I like staff to sit with me at mealtimes and cut up my food because I sometimes choke if I eat too quickly. Please encourage me gently – I eat slowly."*

Practice tip:
If you write a need and can't picture the support happening, it needs more detail.

Using Evidence to Identify Needs

Good care planning is **evidence-based**, not assumption-based.
Use a combination of:

- **Assessments:** falls risk, nutrition, continence, skin integrity.
- **Observations:** changes in behaviour, mobility, appetite.
- **Conversations:** with the person, family, or advocates.
- **Professional input:** GP, District Nurse, SALT, OT, Physiotherapist.

Always ask: *What is this need based on?*
(Links to **CQC E1.1** – evidence-based assessment aligned with **NICE** standards.)

Least Restrictive Practice

When writing about needs, the goal is *support, not control.*
Restrictive:

> *"John should not walk without his frame."*

Least Restrictive:

> *"John sometimes forgets to use his frame. Staff should remind him and supervise to reduce risk of falls. Encourage walking safely so John maintains independence."*

This upholds the **Mental Capacity Act (2005)** principle of *least restriction.*
Legal Reminder:

If a person lacks capacity, decisions must be made in their **best interests** under the MCA.

Where restrictions are required, they must follow the **Liberty Protection Safeguards (LPS)** — the least restrictive option, always reviewed and recorded.

Involving the Person and Family

The best identified needs are **co-produced.**

Families and residents often spot details staff might miss:

> *"Mary's daughter explained she becomes anxious at night, so reassurance is needed then."*
>
> *"Ali told us he needs quiet time after meals, as he feels overwhelmed in busy rooms."*

Co-production ensures accuracy, empathy, and trust.

Life Story and Background

A person is never just a list of tasks — they have a history, personality, and identity.

Examples in practice:

- *Elsie (teacher):* "Elsie values structure. She becomes distressed if her morning routine is disrupted, so staff maintain a consistent order of care."
- *David (farmer):* "David feels calmer outdoors. Staff support him to spend time in the garden daily."
- *Maria (sociable):* "Maria thrives on conversation. Encourage her to attend group activities."

- *Sam (independent):* "Sam values choice. Offer help but allow him to attempt tasks first."

Practice tip:
Even if time is short, ask:

> *"Tell me one thing that really matters to you?"*
> *(This supports* ***NICE QS13*** *– holistic, person-led assessment.)*

Reflection Corner

- Have you seen a plan entry so vague you weren't sure what to do?
- How could it be written more clearly?
- What difference does detail make to dignity and safety?

Pitfalls to Avoid

- Vague wording — always describe *how, when, why,* and *by whom.*
- Jargon — avoid terms like "non-compliant" or "challenging behaviour." Use plain, respectful language.
- Over-generalising — break broad needs into specific situations.
- Copy-and-paste — use the person's own words.
- Out-of-date information — review after any change in health or preference.
- Ignoring voice/family input — co-produce and credit contributors.
- Missing legal checks — apply **MCA** and **LPS** as required.
- Breaching confidentiality — include only information needed for safe care.
- Weak governance — managers must audit the quality of need statements.

Warm Testimony – One Thing I Learned

> *"When I first started caring, I wrote 'needs help with meals.'*
> *A colleague showed me how to add detail about food type, pace, and risks.*
> *I realised clear care plans are about dignity and safety, not just paperwork."*
> *— Senior Carer, 2024*

Quick Practice Checklist

- Is the need **specific** and **evidence-based**?
- Could a new staff member understand exactly what to do?
- Does it reflect the person's **voice and preferences**?
- Does it balance **safety with independence and choice**?

Confidentiality Note

Include only information necessary for safe care.
Store and share securely, following **GDPR** and service policy.

Leadership Link

Managers should review the clarity of identified needs through supervision, audits, and spot checks.
Clear language reduces risk and demonstrates compliance with **CQC Well-Led (W2.1)**.

Activity – Rewrite Vague Needs

Rewrite these in clear, person-centred detail (what, when, why, how, and preferences):

- "Resident needs help with washing."
- "Resident needs help with medication."
- "Resident is forgetful."

Role Reflections

- **Care staff:** Clear needs reduce stress and guesswork.
- **Kitchen teams:** Dining details protect dignity and safety.
- **Laundry teams:** Understanding continence and clothing needs preserves comfort.
- **Maintenance:** Mobility details guide grab rails, lighting, and flooring.

Key Takeaways

- Needs must be clear, specific, and compassionate.
- Cover health, emotional, social, cultural, and spiritual aspects.
- Avoid vague wording and jargon; co-produce with the person and family.
- Balance safety with independence and choice.
- Clear needs make care safer, kinder, and more consistent.

Chapter Summary

The Identified Needs section is the foundation of safe, effective care.

Done well, it guides staff with clarity and empathy.

Done poorly, it creates confusion and risk.

The next step — turning needs into **Aims of the Plan** — transforms support into purpose.

Compliance Spine

- **CQC KLOE:** Effective (E1.1) | Safe (S2.1) | Well-Led (W2.1).
- **NICE QS13:** Assessments include physical, psychological, social, spiritual, cultural, and environmental needs.
- **Audit Question:**
- Would a new staff member, reading this need, know *exactly* what to do and why — while respecting the person's life story and preferences?

End of Chapter 4

Five

From Needs to Aims

Turning Support into Purpose

By now, we've explored how to record someone's **strengths** (what they can do) and **needs** (where they require support).

The next step is to ask:

> *What are we actually working towards through this care and support?*

That's where the **Aim of Plan** comes in.

Strengths, Needs, and Aims – The Connection

Think of it like this:

- **Strengths** – what the person can do.

- **Needs** – where the person requires support.
- **Aim** – the goal or purpose — the *why* behind the care.

Without a clear aim, a plan can feel like a list of chores.

With an aim, it becomes a purposeful, empowering roadmap that makes sense to staff, families, and — most importantly — the person themselves.

Example

Need: John requires support with personal care.

Aim: To support John to remain clean, comfortable, and confident, while maximising his independence in personal hygiene.

Notice how the aim isn't about *washing John* — it's about protecting his **dignity, comfort, and confidence.**

Why Aims Matter

- **For the person:** Aims provide direction, control, and hope.
- **For staff:** They explain *why* each action matters — not just *what* to do.
- **For families:** They reassure that their loved one's dignity and individuality are central.
- **For inspectors:** They show care is outcomes-focused, not task-driven.
- **For everyone:** They promote safe risk-taking, balancing independence with safety.

Without aims, care looks like "wash, dress, feed."

With aims, care looks like "support dignity, encourage independence, promote wellbeing."

The SMART Principle

Aims should always follow the SMART rule:

- **Specific** – clear and focused.
- **Measurable** – you can tell if it's achieved.
- **Achievable** – realistic for the person.
- **Relevant** – meaningful to their life and values.
- **Time-bound** – includes a timeframe, where appropriate.

Example

Vague: "Improve mobility."

SMART:

> *"To support Margaret to safely walk short distances with her frame twice daily, so that she maintains independence and strength while reducing her risk of falls."*

Practice tip:

Add the phrase *"so that..."* when writing an aim — it instantly links the task to a meaningful outcome.

Linking Aims to Life Story and Identity

Aims should reflect who the person is — their history, character, and passions.

Examples:

- **Retired gardener:** "To support John to safely access the garden twice weekly, with staff nearby, so he continues enjoying his passion for plants while reducing fall risks."

- **Lifelong cook:** "To enable Fatima to stay involved in mealtimes by stirring, tasting, or choosing ingredients, so she remains connected to her identity as a cook while staff manage safety."
- **Person of faith:** "To ensure Peter can attend church weekly or access faith services at home, so his spiritual wellbeing is supported safely and reliably."

When aims are linked to life story, they honour individuality, not just routine.

Empowerment Through Aims

Compare the difference:
Task-based:

> *"Ensure meals are provided daily."*

Person-centred:

> *"Support Anna to enjoy regular, balanced meals that meet her diabetic needs, so she feels energised and satisfied."*

One is a tick-box; the other is care with meaning.
Adding *"so that"* turns tasks into empowerment.

Reflection Corner

- Was the aim SMART?
- Did it reflect dignity, independence, or personality?
- Did it include safe risk-taking?
- Would the person or their family recognise themselves in it?

Pitfalls to Avoid

- **Too vague:** "Keep resident safe." (Safe from what? How?)
- **Too clinical:** "Maintain hydration per NICE guidance." (Where's the person's voice?)
- **Too ambitious:** "Help Mary walk independently again" (if her condition makes this impossible).
- **Too restrictive:** "Do not allow Margaret to walk without staff." (Removes independence unnecessarily.)

Balanced aim:

> *"Support Margaret to walk daily with her frame, with staff nearby for reassurance, so she remains active and confident."*

Good aims balance **realism, aspiration, and safe independence.**

Role-Specific Reflections

- **Carers and nurses:** Aims show that personal care protects dignity and guides when to step back.
- **Family carers:** Aims reassure that independence is valued, not restricted.
- **Kitchen teams:** Aims link food to culture, comfort, and pleasure.
- **Laundry and cleaning staff:** Aims connect clean clothing to comfort, dignity, and routine.
- **Maintenance staff:** Aims highlight how adaptations promote independence, not just safety.
- **Managers:** Aims evidence outcomes-focused, risk-balanced, person-centred care for CQC.
- **Volunteers and activity staff:** Aims remind us that activities

should be meaningful, not just scheduled.

Family Testimony

> *"When Dad's aim was written as 'to help him stay confident when moving around the home,' I felt reassured. It showed staff understood his pride in walking with his frame — it wasn't just about falls; it was about confidence."*
>
> *— Family Member, 2024*

Activity – From Needs to SMART Aims

Rewrite these needs into clear, SMART, person-centred aims that include safe risk-taking:

- **Need:** Resident requires assistance with eating.
- **Aim:** Support Mary to enjoy her meals, eating as independently as possible with adapted cutlery, so she feels satisfied and included at mealtimes.
- **Need:** Resident forgets to take medication.
- **Aim:** Support David to take his medication safely and on time each day, with prompts and supervision, so he remains well and reassured.
- **Need:** Resident becomes anxious in the evening.
- **Aim:** Help Anna feel calm and reassured in the evenings through a consistent routine, soothing music, and staff presence when needed.
- **Need:** Resident is at risk of falls when walking.
- **Aim:** Enable Margaret to continue enjoying daily garden walks with her frame, with staff nearby for reassurance, so she remains active and confident while reducing fall risks.

DoLS / LPS – Protecting Liberty and Rights within Aims

When a person's freedom or choices are restricted for safety, this must always be done with respect and legal protection.

- **DoLS (Deprivation of Liberty Safeguards):** Protects people in care homes or hospitals who lack capacity to consent to certain arrangements.
- **LPS (Liberty Protection Safeguards):** Will soon replace DoLS, expanding protection to all care settings, including community care.

In practice:

When writing aims that include supervision, locked doors, or restricted access, clearly show how the plan:

1. Promotes the **least restrictive** approach possible.
2. Records the **reason and authorisation** (DoLS or LPS).
3. Balances **safety with dignity and independence.**

This demonstrates compliance with **CQC Safe (S2.1)** and **Caring (C1.1)** standards.

DoLS/LPS Mini-Check for Aims:

- Does the aim show how choice and safety are balanced?
- Has the restriction been explained and authorised?
- Is the focus still on independence, not control?

Confidentiality Note

Aims should include only information necessary for safe, effective care.

Personal details must be stored securely and shared only with those directly involved, in line with **GDPR** and confidentiality policy.

Leadership Link

Managers should review the quality of aims during supervision and training.

SMART, person-centred aims provide strong evidence for **CQC Well-Led (W2.1)** and **Effective (E1.4)** standards.

Key Takeaways

- Aims transform needs into purposeful goals.
- SMART principles keep them clear, realistic, and measurable.
- The best aims reflect the person's voice and life story.
- Aims must include safe risk-taking and lawful restriction where needed.
- They turn *tasks* into *care that truly matters.*

Chapter Summary

The **Aim of the Plan** gives care its purpose — showing what we're working towards, why it matters, and how it benefits the person.

Aims should always be SMART, person-centred, and grounded in life story and preference, balancing independence with safety.

When restrictions are necessary, lawful authorisation under **DoLS or LPS** ensures care remains protective, proportionate, and focused on freedom wherever possible.

Next, in Chapter 6, we'll create the **Plan of Action** – the practical steps that bring each aim to life every day.

Compliance Spine

- **CQC KLOE:** Effective (E1.4) | Caring (C1.1) | Responsive (R1.2) | Safe (S2.1) | Well-Led (W2.1).
- **NICE Quality Standard Check:** Are aims SMART, outcomes-focused, and written in the person's voice while supporting safe independence?

Mini-Audit for Staff:

- Does the aim show what we're working towards and why it matters?
- Does it reflect the person's voice and independence?
- Would the person or family recognise themselves in it?
- If liberty is restricted, is it lawful, reviewed, and the least restrictive possible?

End of Chapter 5

Six

Plan of Action

From Aims to Actions: Where Plans Come to Life

Turning Words into Care

Every plan becomes real in the small moments of daily care — a steady hand, a calm tone, or a respectful pause before offering help.

The **Plan of Action** is where the paper plan turns into real, compassionate practice.

It tells everyone how to support the person **safely, consistently, and with dignity** — whether you're a carer, volunteer, nurse, or visiting professional.

> *The* Aim *tells us what we want to achieve.*
> *The* Plan of Action *explains how we make it happen.*

Think of it like a recipe: clear, step-by-step, and detailed enough that anyone can follow it confidently.

A vague instruction such as *"assist with meals"* is like writing *"make food"* in a cookbook — not much help to anyone.

Why Detail Matters

A strong Plan of Action ensures:

- **Consistency:** Everyone supports the resident in the same respectful way.
- **Clarity:** Everyone understands what to do and when.
- **Safety:** Risks are managed, and competence is proven.
- **Dignity and independence:** Choices and routines are honoured.
- **Rights and compliance:** MCA, DoLS/LPS, and safeguarding principles are embedded.
- **Well-led practice:** Each action links to the training and skills required.

Simple Rule

- If the person **can decide**, record their preference.
- If they **cannot**, record how staff will support them in their *Best Interests* — always using the *least-restrictive* option.

Confidentiality Note

Only record information relevant to care.

Handle personal details respectfully, store securely, and share only with those who need to know, in line with **GDPR** and data protection law.

DoLS / LPS – Safeguarding Liberty and Choice

When a person's freedom of movement or decision-making is restricted to keep them safe, this must be **lawful, necessary, and proportionate.**

- **DoLS (Deprivation of Liberty Safeguards):** Protects people in care homes or hospitals who lack capacity to consent to their care.
- **LPS (Liberty Protection Safeguards):** Will replace DoLS, extending protections across all care settings.

If a Plan of Action includes **constant supervision, locked doors, restricted access, or observation**, it must clearly show:

1. **Why** the restriction is needed (the risk and purpose).
2. That the **least-restrictive** option has been chosen.
3. The **legal authorisation** (DoLS now, LPS in future).
4. **How and when** the restriction will be reviewed.

DoLS/LPS Quick Check (for any plan):

- Has capacity been assessed and recorded for this decision?
- Is the least-restrictive option described?
- Is authorisation in place, with a review date recorded?

This demonstrates compliance with **CQC Safe (S2.1)** and **Caring (C1.1)** standards.

Writing Clear, Carer-Friendly Actions

Good Plans of Action are:

- **Step-by-step:** first, next, last.
- **Specific:** include times, equipment, and preferences.
- **Person-centred:** reflect life story, values, and personality.
- **Encouraging:** promote independence and safe risk-taking.
- **Training-linked:** identify skills required for safe delivery.

Example – Personal Care

Poor:

> *"Help resident wash."*

Professional voice:

> *"Support Mary with her morning shower after breakfast. Offer her lavender body wash (her preference). Encourage her to wash her face and arms independently. Assist with her back and legs, keeping her covered with a towel for privacy. Mary enjoys talking about her years in a flower shop — chat about flowers to create a calm, friendly atmosphere. Mary has capacity for this choice and consents to a daily shower. Staff must have completed Personal Care and Dignity Training."*

Person's voice:

> *"I like to shower in the morning after breakfast. Please offer me my lavender body wash and encourage me to wash my face and*

arms myself. I'm happy for you to help with my back and legs but keep me covered with a towel for dignity. I enjoy talking about flowers — please chat with me about my years in the flower shop. I choose to shower daily."

Embedding Life Story, Personality, and Safe Risk-Taking

Plans should show **not just what we do, but who the person is.** Include:

- **Life story:** past roles, hobbies, and achievements.
- **Personality:** gentle, proud, humorous, chatty.
- **Preferences:** food, clothing, music, culture, faith, and routine.
- **Safe risk-taking:** balancing choice and safety.
- **Staff competence:** match support to training.

Example – Mobility
Poor: "Help with mobility."
Good:

"Support Alan to walk from his bedroom to the lounge before lunch. Offer his walking frame and check footwear. Walk beside him at his pace, using positive words for encouragement. Allow him to rest halfway. Alan used to be a football coach — cheer him on like one of his players. Staff must have completed Moving and Handling and Falls Awareness training."

Using SMART in Action Plans

Each action should be **SMART** — Specific, Measurable, Achievable, Relevant, and Time-bound.

Examples:

- *Specific:* "Offer lavender body wash," not "assist with wash."
- *Measurable:* "Encourage Alan to walk daily before lunch."
- *Achievable:* "Short, supported walks."
- *Relevant:* "Supports independence and confidence."
- *Time-bound:* "Daily, reviewed every month."

Practice tip:

Ask yourself:

> *"If I were new to the team, could I follow this plan safely and kindly?"*

Linking to Person-Centred Tools

Use **Helen Sanderson** tools to bring actions to life:

- **One-Page Profiles:** Summarise what's important to and for the person.
- **Important To/For Charts:** Balance wellbeing and safety.
- **Decision-Making Profiles:** Show how much support someone needs with choices.
- **Doughnut Tool:** Identify what must happen versus where staff can adapt for choice.

These tools keep actions personal and empower staff to respond thoughtfully.

Reflection Corner

- Does the Plan of Action describe clear, step-by-step guidance?
- Does it reflect the person's life story and preferences?
- Does it promote independence and safe risk-taking?
- Have training requirements been listed?
- Would this plan meet CQC standards for Safe, Caring, and Well-Led practice?

Testimony

> *"Before, our plans just said 'assist with meals'. I never knew what that really meant.*
>
> *Now we include food preferences, risks, and conversation ideas — residents are happier, and I feel more confident."*
>
> *— Care Worker, Residential Home, 2024*

Activity – Rewrite Poor Statements

Poor: "Assist with medication."

Improved:

> *"Support Mrs Khan with her 9 a.m. tablets. Prompt her to take them with water and check she has swallowed safely. Record on the MAR chart. Mrs Khan chooses to take her medicine in the lounge with tea. Staff must have Medication Awareness training."*

Poor: "Help with mobility."

Improved:

> *"Support Alan to walk from his bedroom to the lounge before lunch. Offer his walking frame, check footwear, and walk beside him. Allow him to rest halfway. Staff must have Moving and Handling and Falls Awareness training."*

Poor: "Support at mealtimes."
Improved:

> *"Encourage James to eat lunch in the dining room with friends. Cut food into small pieces, provide thickened fluids per SALT guidance, and sit with him for reassurance. James enjoys talking about football — chat about his favourite team. Staff must have Dysphagia Awareness and Food Hygiene training."*

Role-Specific Reflections

- **Kitchen teams:** Do meal plans promote dignity and choice?
- **Laundry staff:** Are clothing and linen handled respectfully?
- **Maintenance:** Are walking routes safe, with good lighting and rails?
- **Managers:** Can you evidence staff competence for each action?
- **Carers:** Do daily actions match what's written in the plan?

Pitfalls to Avoid

- Using vague wording like "assist with…"
- Forgetting to link actions to training.
- Ignoring preferences, personality, or dignity.
- Removing independence instead of encouraging it.
- Adding unnecessary personal details that breach confidentiality.
- Copying and pasting identical instructions for multiple residents.

Leadership Link

Managers must ensure every action is written, taught, and reviewed through supervision.

Clear, person-centred actions demonstrate competence under **CQC Well-Led (W2.1)** and **Safe (S2.1)** standards.

Compliance Spine

- **CQC Quality Statements:**
- Safe (S2.1) — Actions promote safety and choice.
- Effective (E1.4) — Steps achieve planned aims.
- Caring (C1.1) — Residents treated with respect and compassion.
- Responsive (R1.2) — Plans adapt to individual needs.
- Well-Led (W2.1) — Leaders ensure staff competence.
- **NICE Standards (QS194 & NG108):**
- Start by assuming capacity.
- Record wishes and preferences clearly.
- Use Best-Interest decisions only when capacity is lacking.
- Encourage safe independence wherever possible.

Manager's Mini-Audit Prompt:

Can you show that every action is clear, person-centred, rights-aware (MCA/DoLS/LPS), and carried out only by trained staff?

Key Takeaways

- Plans of Action turn aims into daily steps.
- Actions must be clear, person-centred, and safe.
- Life story and personality make care meaningful.
- Training links prove competence.

- Safe risk-taking promotes dignity and independence.
- MCA, DoLS, and least-restrictive principles guide every step.

Chapter Summary

The **Plan of Action** is where care planning becomes real.

It turns good intentions into compassionate, skilled care that every team member can follow confidently.

When actions reflect **life story, preferences, legal safeguards (MCA/DoLS/LPS), and staff competence**, they don't just meet CQC standards —

they **improve real lives.**

> *Clear actions make care safe.*
> *Compassionate actions make care meaningful.*

End of Chapter 6

Seven

Desired Outcomes

The Heart of Every Plan

Every Plan Has a Purpose

Every care plan is a promise of progress — a story of where we are now and where we hope to be next.

The **Desired Outcome** is that hopeful point on the horizon — the target we're working toward with the person.

If the **Plan of Action** is the route, then the **Desired Outcome** is the destination.

What "Desired Outcome" Really Means

A **Desired Outcome** describes what we want to happen *as a result* of our support — the improvement, confidence, or comfort the person should achieve.

It is not what's happening now; it's what we are **working towards.** A clear outcome brings direction, hope, and accountability.

Why It Matters

- Keeps the plan **purposeful** rather than task-based.
- Gives the person a clear goal to work toward.
- Helps carers measure progress and celebrate success.
- Shows CQC that care is **planned, reviewed, and effective.**
- Encourages dignity, independence, and safe risk-taking.

When outcomes are clear, care has meaning.

How to Write a Desired Outcome

A good outcome is:

- **Future-focused:** describes what will change or improve.
- **Person-centred:** reflects the person's wishes.
- **Positive:** shows what we're achieving, not just avoiding.
- **SMART:** Specific, Measurable, Achievable, Relevant, Time-bound.

Examples (written in future tense):

- For Mary to walk with her frame confidently and safely.
- For Ali to maintain a healthy weight and enjoy his meals.
- For Anna to settle calmly at night and sleep through most evenings.
- For Elsie to video-call her grandchildren every Sunday.

From Aims to Outcomes

Here's how the flow connects:

Current Strengths: Mary can walk short distances with her frame.

Identified Need: She needs support with balance and confidence.

Aim of the Plan: To help Mary maintain independence when walking.

Plan of Action: Staff check footwear, supervise, and encourage daily walks.

Desired Outcome: For Mary to walk with her frame confidently and safely, maintaining independence and reducing falls risk.

Write Desired Outcomes as if you're describing success after the plan has worked.

Writing SMART Desired Outcomes

Specific: For Alan to walk to the lounge daily using his frame.

Measurable: To complete this four times a week without falls.

Achievable: Short walks with rests.

Relevant: Linked to Alan's wish to stay active.

Time-bound: To be achieved within one month and reviewed.

SMART outcomes turn abstract goals into practical progress.

Examples Across Domains

- **Physical:** For Margaret to maintain safe mobility with her frame twice daily.
- **Emotional:** For Anna to feel calmer by bedtime within two weeks.
- **Social:** For John to join the gardening club twice a week.
- **Nutritional:** For Ali to maintain a stable weight over the next month.

Each one is personal, measurable, and focused on wellbeing.

Legal and Ethical Considerations

If a person lacks capacity to set their own goals, outcomes must reflect **Best Interests** decisions under the **Mental Capacity Act (2005)** and use the **least-restrictive option.**

All outcomes should:

- Protect dignity and choice.
- Support safe independence.
- Be reviewed regularly for relevance and accuracy.

DoLS / LPS – Safeguarding Liberty and Choice

When freedom of movement or decision-making is restricted for safety, it must always be lawful and proportionate.

- **DoLS (Deprivation of Liberty Safeguards):** Apply in care homes or hospitals when a person lacks capacity to consent to their care.
- **LPS (Liberty Protection Safeguards):** Will soon replace DoLS, expanding protection across all care settings.

In practice:

If a care plan includes supervision, locked doors, or restricted access, record:

1. **Why** the restriction is needed.
2. **How** it promotes safety and wellbeing.
3. That it is the **least restrictive** option.
4. **When** it will be reviewed.

These safeguards show compliance with **CQC Safe (S2.1)** and **Caring (C1.1)** standards — protecting both rights and safety.

Confidentiality Note

Record only information relevant to care.
Store and share securely in line with **GDPR** and service policy.

Person-Centred Tools to Shape Outcomes

Use practical tools to co-produce meaningful targets:

- **One-Page Profile:** What is important *to* and *for* the person.
- **Decision-Making Profile:** Which decisions the person makes and where support is needed.
- **Doughnut Tool:** What must happen versus what can flex for choice.

Toolkit tip:
Keep these tools beside you when writing outcomes — they make every target unique and human.

Writing in the Right Voice

- **Resident's voice:** "I want to walk safely and confidently with my frame."
- **Professional voice:** "For Mary to walk safely and confidently with her frame."

Best practice:
Include both — the resident's for identity, the professional's for clarity.

Start each outcome with "For [Name] to..." to keep it future-focused.

Reflection Corner

- Are the outcomes realistic targets, not completed results?
- Would the person recognise these as their own goals?
- Do they encourage dignity, choice, and independence?
- Can progress be evidenced during review?

Testimony

> *"When we started writing outcomes as clear targets, reviews made sense — we could see real progress and celebrate it."*
> *— Senior Carer, Residential Home, 2024*

Activity – Rewrite Vague Statements as SMART Targets

Poor: "Resident to stay safe."

SMART: For John to walk safely using his frame each day with supervision for reassurance, to be achieved within one month.

Poor: "Resident to eat well."

SMART: For Mary to eat at least 75% of her meals daily with encouragement, maintaining weight over four weeks.

Poor: "Resident to join activities."

SMART: For Amira to attend her chosen art session twice weekly within one month.

Poor: "Resident to improve mobility."

SMART: For Paul to walk to the dining room each day with staff encouragement, maintaining confidence over six weeks.

Pitfalls to Avoid

- Vague language like "stay safe" — specify what that means.
- Task-lists disguised as outcomes — "provide meals" is not a target.
- Over-ambitious or unrealistic goals.
- Over-restrictive wording that removes independence.
- Missing review dates or follow-up.
- Skipping MCA or LPS checks where capacity is in doubt.
- Copy-and-paste goals — every person's outcome should feel personal.

Role-Specific Reflection Box

- **Carers and nurses:** Do outcomes show what success looks like in daily life?
- **Families:** Do they reflect genuine goals and preferences?
- **Kitchen teams:** How do menus support nutritional outcomes?
- **Laundry and housekeeping:** Does presentation help residents feel confident?
- **Maintenance:** Do adaptations support independence?
- **Managers:** Can you evidence how targets link to reviews and audits?
- **Activities staff:** Are social outcomes meaningful, inclusive, and measurable?

Leadership Link

Leaders should audit outcomes regularly through supervision and reviews.

Ask: *Are they SMART, person-centred, and being tracked?*

This demonstrates compliance with **CQC Well-Led (W2.1)** and supports **Effective (E1.4)** and **Responsive (R1.2)** practice.

Compliance Spine

- **CQC Quality Statements:**
- Safe (S2.1): Targets promote safety and choice.
- Effective (E1.4): Outcomes define what improvement looks like.
- Caring (C1.1): Goals respect dignity and individuality.
- Responsive (R1.2): Outcomes are personal and reviewable.
- Well-Led (W2.1): Leaders ensure targets guide daily practice.
- **NICE Standards (QS13, QS194):**
- Focus on quality of life, not just clinical change.
- Agree outcomes with residents or representatives.
- Review and adapt when needs or wishes change.

Manager's Mini-Audit Prompt:

Can you show that every Desired Outcome is realistic, measurable, co-produced, and reviewed on schedule?

Key Takeaways

- Desired Outcomes are **targets**, not results.
- They describe what success looks like when the plan works.
- SMART outcomes make care measurable and reviewable.
- Person-centred tools bring outcomes to life.
- Each outcome should reflect **dignity, choice, and independence.**
- Reviews turn targets into achievements.

Chapter Summary

The **Desired Outcome** is the target — a clear picture of what you and the person are working toward.

It keeps the plan alive, hopeful, and measurable.

Each target should build independence, protect dignity, and celebrate individuality.

When restrictions are necessary, lawful authorisation under **DoLS or LPS** ensures they remain safe, justified, and regularly reviewed.

> *A clear Desired Outcome turns a care plan from a list of tasks into a promise of change.*

End of Chapter 7

Eight

From Paper to Practice: Making Care Plans Come Alive

The Journey So Far

Across these chapters, we've built every part of a strong, person-centred care plan — from **strengths** and **needs**, to **aims**, **actions**, and **desired outcomes**.

Now, as we close, remember this:

A care plan is never just paperwork.

It is a *living agreement* between a person, their loved ones, and the team that supports them.

The best plans don't sit in folders — they live in **daily routines, conversations, and smiles.**

The Complete Care-Planning Spine

Every great plan follows this golden thread:

1. **Current Strengths / Abilities** – Start with what the person can do.
2. *"Mary can walk short distances with her frame."*
3. **Identified Needs** – Describe where support is required.
4. *"Mary needs supervision for balance and confidence."*
5. **Aim of the Plan** – Explain what we hope to achieve.
6. *"To help Mary maintain independence when walking."*
7. **Plan of Action** – Detail the step-by-step support.
8. *"Staff to check footwear, supervise, and encourage daily walks."*
9. **Desired Outcome** – Show the goal we're working toward.
10. *"For Mary to walk with her frame confidently and safely."*

When these stages connect, care becomes purposeful, personal, and measurable.

It moves from **tasks** to **stories** — from doing *for* someone to doing *with* them.

From Plan to Practice

Once a plan is written, people bring it to life.

Every role plays a part in turning words into wellbeing:

- **Carers:** bring compassion and presence.
- **Kitchen teams:** bring nourishment, culture, and comfort.
- **Laundry staff:** protect dignity through clean, familiar clothing.
- **Maintenance teams:** make spaces safe and accessible.
- **Managers and leaders:** ensure clarity, consistency, and reflection.

When everyone connects to the plan, people feel **comfort, confidence, and continuity.**

Practice Tip:

During handover, link your updates to the plan —

> *"We supported Mary's garden walk today; she used her frame confidently."*

Staying Compliant, Staying Human

CQC Quality Statements

- **Safe (S2.1):** Residents live safely while maintaining independence.
- **Effective (E1.4):** Plans achieve meaningful, measurable results.
- **Caring (C1.1):** Every decision upholds dignity and respect.
- **Responsive (R1.2):** Plans reflect preferences and are reviewed regularly.
- **Well-Led (W2.1):** Leaders ensure plans guide daily practice.

NICE Guidance (QS13, QS194)

- Base care on what matters most to the person.
- Always assume capacity first.
- If capacity is lacking, act in **Best Interests**.
- Review regularly and record outcomes clearly.

MCA Reminder

If a person lacks capacity, involve family or advocates, use the **least restrictive option**, and clearly record your reasoning and review dates.

Every decision should protect both **safety** and **freedom** — in equal measure.

DoLS / LPS – Protecting Liberty and Rights

When someone's freedom of movement or choice is restricted for safety, this must always be **lawful, proportionate, and respectful.**

- **DoLS (Deprivation of Liberty Safeguards):** Protect people in care homes or hospitals who lack capacity to consent to their care.
- **LPS (Liberty Protection Safeguards):** Will replace DoLS, creating a simpler, more inclusive framework across all care settings.

In practice, if a plan includes **supervision, locked doors, or restricted movement**, record:

1. The **reason** for the restriction.
2. How it **promotes safety and wellbeing.**
3. That the **least-restrictive** option was chosen.
4. How and when it will be **reviewed.**

This protects both **rights and compliance** under **CQC Safe (S2.1)** and **Caring (C1.1).**

Confidentiality Note

Care plans must include only information necessary for safe, effective support.

Store and share them securely, in line with **GDPR** and service policy.

Reflection Corner

Ask yourself and your team:

- Do our plans feel alive and personal?
- Do our daily actions connect to each person's goals?
- Do reviews celebrate progress and learning?
- Would a CQC inspector see people and purpose — not just paperwork?

> *"A good plan changes as the person's life does — it grows, just like they do."*
> *— Deputy Manager, Care Home, 2024*

Practice in Action – Keeping Plans Alive

- Read one plan a day and reconnect with what matters most.
- Involve the person in every review and update.
- Share insights at handovers to maintain consistency.
- Celebrate progress — even small wins matter.
- Update promptly when needs, wishes, or health change.

Leadership Link

Managers should model reflective practice and ask during supervision:

> *"How have you brought someone's plan to life this week?"*

This builds a culture of **living care**, not just compliant care.

Compliance Spine – Final Reflection

- **Strengths-Based (Caring / Responsive):** Recognises who residents are, not just what they need.
- **Empowering (Effective):** Residents achieve goals that matter to them.
- **Dignity and Independence (Caring):** Every plan promotes choice and control.
- **Safe Risk-Taking (Safe / Well-Led):** Balances safety with freedom.
- **Person-Centred (Responsive):** Plans are unique, meaningful, and regularly reviewed.

DoLS / LPS Quick Audit Checklist

For every plan that includes supervision, restricted movement, or environmental safety measures:

1. **Capacity Check:** Has capacity been assessed and recorded for this specific decision?
2. **Least-Restrictive Principle:** Have we shown how independence and choice are promoted, with restrictions minimised?
3. **Authorisation and Review:** Is authorisation in place under DoLS (or future LPS), and is the review date recorded?

If you answer *no* to any of these, discuss it with your manager or Best Interests Assessor.

The goal is always to protect both **rights and safety.**

Key Takeaways

- Every plan begins with a person's story.
- Desired Outcomes are the shared goals that keep care focused.
- Actions make those goals real, step by step.
- Collaboration turns paperwork into partnership.
- Compassion creates compliance — when care feels human, it meets every standard.
- A living plan is the heartbeat of quality care — reviewed, refreshed, and always about the person first.

Chapter Summary

A great care plan is not a form — it is a *shared story of support.*

It connects what matters **to** the person with what matters **for** their safety.

When we write clearly, act consistently, and review reflectively, care becomes both **compliant and compassionate.**

Plans that live through people's actions become the strongest evidence of quality care:

safe, kind, and individual.

Care planning is not paperwork — it's person-work.

End of Chapter 8

Nine

Dedication & Closing Reflections

Dedication – For Everyone Who Brings Care to Life

This book is dedicated to everyone who gives care with heart and purpose — in homes, hospitals, care homes, supported living, and family homes across the country.

To the **carers and nurses** who show up each day with patience, skill, and compassion — your hands do more than complete tasks; they bring comfort, dignity, and safety.

To the **kitchen teams**, whose meals nourish more than bodies — they feed memories, culture, and connection.

To the **laundry and housekeeping teams**, who protect dignity quietly — through the soft feel of clean clothes and the familiar scent of home.

To the **maintenance staff**, who keep spaces safe and welcoming — every working light and sturdy rail says, *"You matter."*

To the **managers and leaders**, who turn policy into culture — thank you for making compassion measurable and compliance meaningful.

To the **families and friends**, who trust, advocate, and love through every change — your insight and care are the heartbeat of true partnership.

To the **residents and people we support** — thank you for teaching us what matters most. Your stories shape the soul of care planning: courage, humour, love, and resilience.

And finally, to every **learner and leader** who chooses to make care plans person-centred, empowering, and kind — you are changing care for good.

Final Reflection

A care plan is never just a document — it is a story, a safeguard, and a promise.

Each plan quietly says:

> *"I see you."*
> *"I value you."*
> *"I will support you to live your life, your way."*

That is the true heart of compassionate care.

With Gratitude

Written with love and respect for all who care —
in every role, every setting, every day.

End of Dedication

Ten

References and Resources

These trusted UK organisations and frameworks support the compassionate, person-centred principles shared throughout Writing Lives, Not Just Plans – A Compassionate Guide to Person-Centred Care Planning.

Each link offers free, practical resources for carers, families, and professionals dedicated to making care more personal, safe, and empowering.

Care Quality Commission (CQC)

🔗 www.cqc.org.uk

Guidance on the five key questions — *Safe, Effective, Caring, Responsive,* and *Well-Led* — and the Quality Statements that define good care.

Use this site to check your service's compliance, inspection reports, and person-centred practice standards.

NICE – National Institute for Health and Care Excellence

🔗 www.nice.org.uk

Evidence-based quality standards and clinical guidance for safe, effective, person-centred care.

Key standards include:

- **QS13** – End-of-Life Care for People with Dementia
- **QS194** – Supporting Adult Social Care

These standards help align care plans with nationally recognised benchmarks of best practice.

SCIE – Social Care Institute for Excellence

🔗 www.scie.org.uk

Free toolkits, videos, and case studies on strengths-based and person-centred care.

A valuable source for reflective learning, leadership development, and supervision materials.

Helen Sanderson Associates (HSA)

🔗 www.helensanderson.net

Creators of the **person-centred thinking tools** featured throughout this guide, including:

- One-Page Profiles
- Important To/Important For Charts
- Decision-Making Profiles
- Doughnut Tools

These tools help balance individuality, safety, and independence in care planning.

Skills for Care

🔗 www.skillsforcare.org.uk
Provides workforce development frameworks, training standards, and leadership support for adult social care.
A practical resource for managers, carers, and teams working to meet CQC and regulatory expectations.

Alzheimer's Society (UK)

🔗 www.alzheimers.org.uk
Offers practical guidance and emotional support for people living with dementia and their carers.
Use this site for up-to-date information on communication, wellbeing, and dementia-inclusive care.

NHS England – Personalised Care

🔗 www.england.nhs.uk/personalisedcare
National guidance on personalised care, shared decision-making, and person-centred planning across health and social care systems.
Helps align care plans with the NHS's broader personalised care goals.

DoLS and LPS – Safeguarding Liberty and Rights

🔗 www.gov.uk/dols | www.gov.uk/liberty-protection-safeguards
The **Deprivation of Liberty Safeguards (DoLS)** and the upcoming **Liberty Protection Safeguards (LPS)** protect people who may lack

mental capacity to make certain decisions.

They ensure that any restrictions on freedom are lawful, proportionate, and in the person's best interests.

Every care plan that includes supervision, locked doors, or restricted access should:

- reference these safeguards,
- show least-restrictive practice, and
- include review dates.

💡 *Tip:* Use your care plan to demonstrate how freedom, dignity, and safety are balanced every day.

Reflective Practice Favourites

- *What's Working / Not Working* – Helen Sanderson Associates reflection tool.
- *Positive and Productive Meetings* – SCIE guide for involving residents and families.
- *The Six Cs of Nursing* – Care, Compassion, Competence, Communication, Courage, and Commitment.

These frameworks remind us that paperwork only becomes powerful when it changes lives.

Citation Note

All referenced frameworks and tools are credited to their original creators (CQC, NICE, HSA, SCIE, Skills for Care, Alzheimer's Society, NHS England, and DoLS/LPS guidance).

This book adapts them for educational and training purposes within the context of person-centred care planning.

Final Reflection

Every policy, tool, and standard exists for one reason —
to help people live their chosen lives with dignity, safety, and joy.

End of References and Resources

About the Author

About the Author

Dennis Cal-Ortiz Pantua has spent more than two decades in the care community — from hands-on support to leadership, mentoring, and writing.

He has worked alongside carers, nurses, GPs, managers, families, kitchen teams, and volunteers, liaising closely with mental health teams and helping everyone see how their role makes a real difference to someone's daily life.

His passion lies in transforming care documents into person-centred narratives that honour individuality, foster independence, and uphold dignity.

Dennis combines professional expertise with a deep respect for the humanity behind every care plan.

His writing reflects the principles of the Care Quality Commission (CQC) and NICE Quality Standards, translated into plain, compassionate English so that everyone — from new carers to registered managers — can use them confidently in daily practice.

"I've seen how a few well-chosen words can transform care.

A good plan doesn't just record what we do — it reminds us why we care."

Through his experience, training, consultancy, and writing, Dennis continues to support the care homes he works with to build confident, person-centred teams that value safe risk-taking, independence, and inclusion.

His approach is simple but powerful: kindness, clarity, and consistency.

www.ingramcontent.com/pod-product-compliance
Lightning Source LLC
LaVergne TN
LVHW090426210926
848480LV00002B/702